The WONDERFUL CHRISTMAS UNDIES

HarperCollins*Publishers*
77–85 Fulham Palace Road,
Hammersmith, London W6 8JB

www.harpercollins.co.uk

First published by HarperCollins*Publishers* 2008
1

A catalogue record of this book
is available from the British Library

ISBN-13 978 0 00 728145 9

Printed and bound in China by Leo Paper Products Limited

The WONDERFUL CHRISTMAS UNDIES

Such is the RADIANCE of her BEAUTY that she hides behind the giant potato for fear of dazzling the mortals

The BEAUTIFUL CHRISTMAS ANGEL

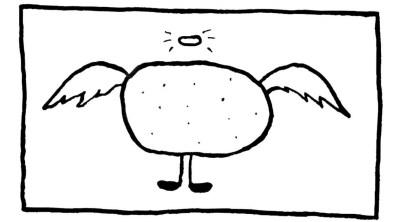

The LOVELY SNOWFLAKES

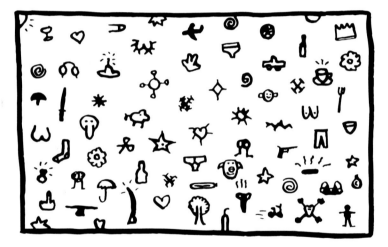

They SAY that every Snowflake is a DIFFERENT shape. But how do they KNOW? who CHECKS?

Whoever used to check is probably in the BONKERS HOUSE by now

NAMES of my BRUSSELS SPROUTS
(including OBSERVATIONS about them)

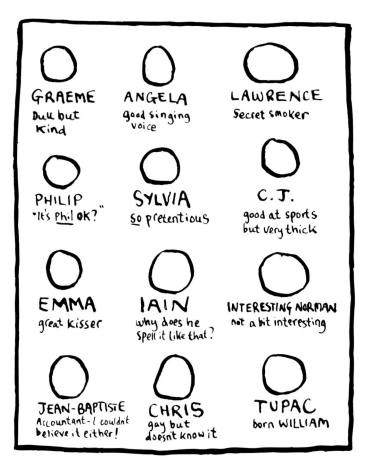

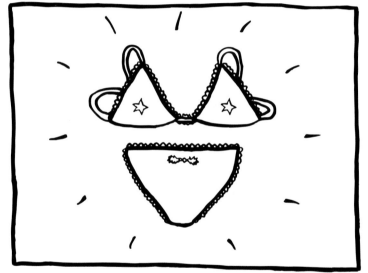

So powerful was their spell that ladies SIGHED with PLEASURE at their beauty and grown men fell to their knees and WEPT

And in his heavy sack
The big man carried
GLORY, WONDER,
HAPPINESS and LOVE

SANTA'S HEAVY SACK

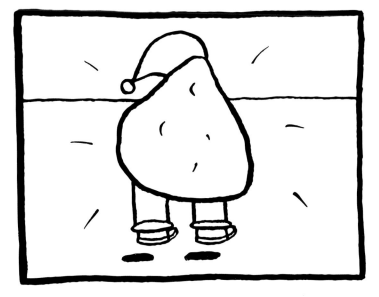

SAUSAGE of PEACE

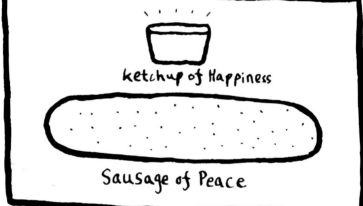

ketchup of Happiness

Sausage of Peace

May the SAUSAGE of PEACE
forever be dipped in the
KETCHUP of HAPPINESS

At Christmas let us **PRAISE** the television for all the **WORLDLY JOY** it brings mankind

CHRISTMAS TELEVISION

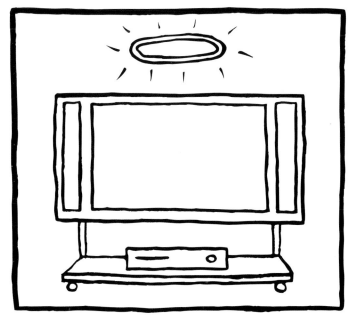

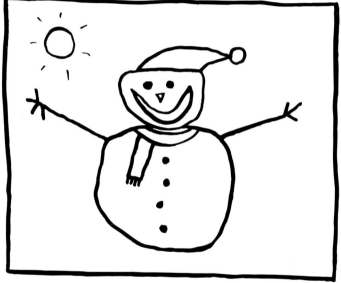

May the HAPPINESS of
the Happy Snowman never
melt in the WARM and
LOVELY garden of your
HEART

They say that with a present it's the
THOUGHT that counts. So this year
I am going to **THINK** for you a brand
new **DIAMOND** necklace.

Generous Thought

If it works, I promise to get you matching
earrings next year as well!!

MY CHRISTMAS EXPERIMENT

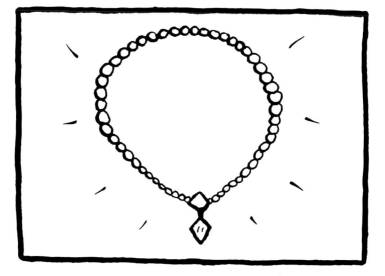

The CHRISTMAS CAKE of LIFE

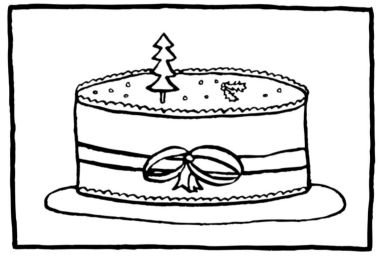

May you always find the ICING
on the Christmas Cake of LIFE

1. Vol au Vent of LOVE

2. Stuffing Ball of PEACE

3. Hazelnut of HARMONY

4. Cocktail Sausage of HAPPINESS

CHRISTMAS SNACK ASSORTMENT

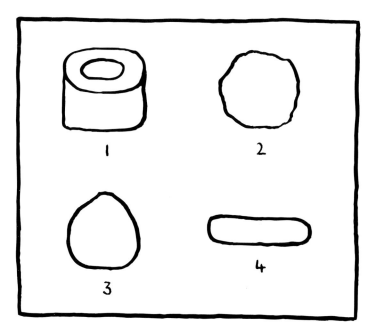

A CHRISTMAS WISH

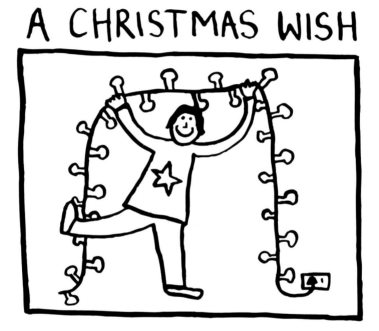

May each twinkling light be a HOPE of yours for the FUTURE. And for each one that blows may there be a BRIGHTER and more BEAUTIFUL bulb in the glorious Trouser Pocket of FORTUNE

His TASTE may be BITTER
but his NOURISHMENT is SWEET.

Lesson to Learn

As with Iain - so with LIFE

IAIN the BRUSSELS SPROUT

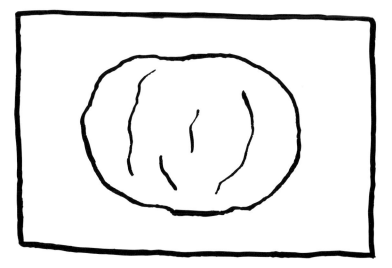

CHRISTMAS HAPPINESS

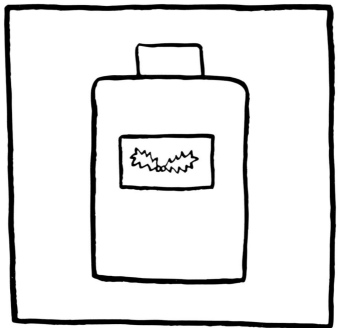

Directions for Use

Apply liberally to face and body for everlasting JOY

THE END